Medical
Tourism

An Easy And Concise Book For Medical Tourism

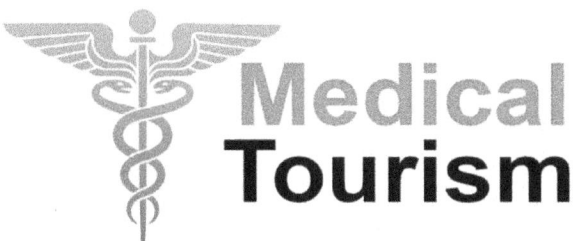

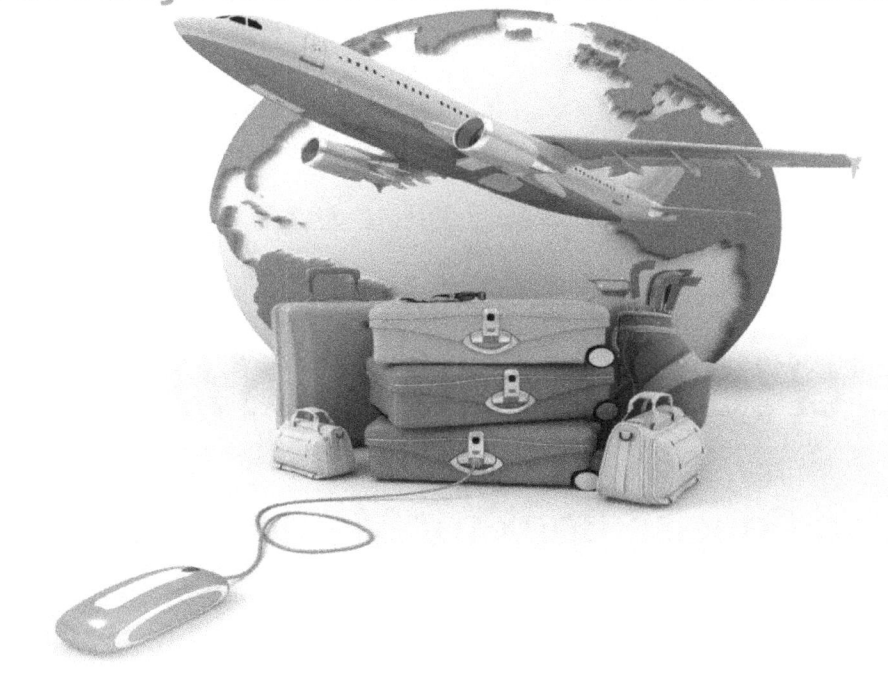

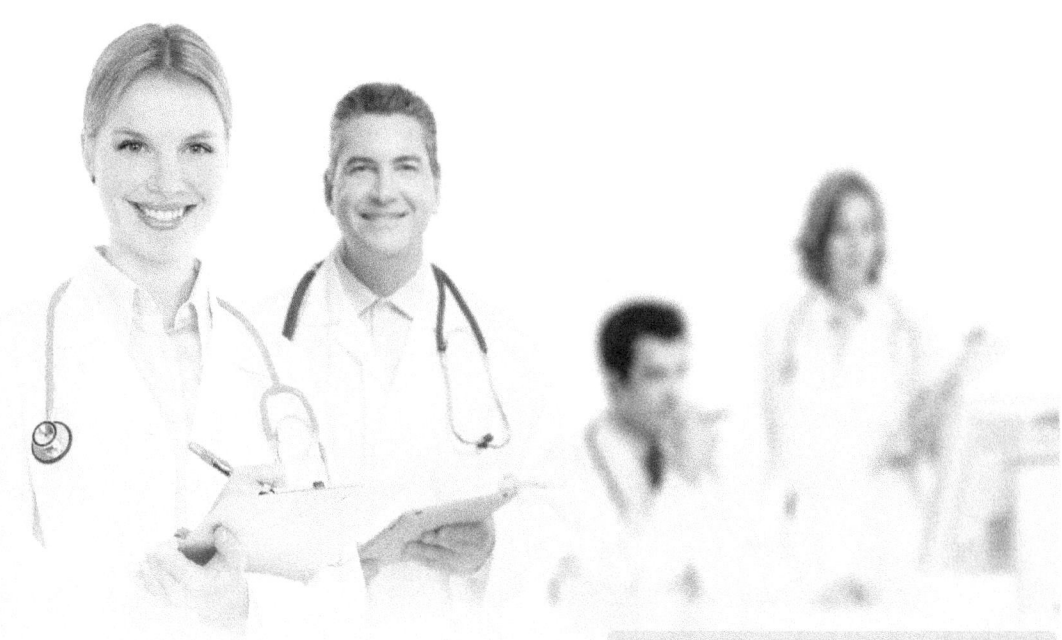

Vindimear D Heart

Medical Tourism

An Easy and Concise Book for Medical Tourism

Table of Contents:

Introduction   3-5
History of medical tourism   6-14
How to plan your medical tourism   15-18
Important steps to plan medical tour   19-21
What to do during stay abroad   22-24
What to do after reaching home   25-26
How to make your journey valuable   27
Important steps to make your journey value   28-29
Country with highest medical tourism   30-45
Advantage of Medical Tourism   46-47
Disadvantage of Medical Tourism   48
Conclusion   49-50

Introduction

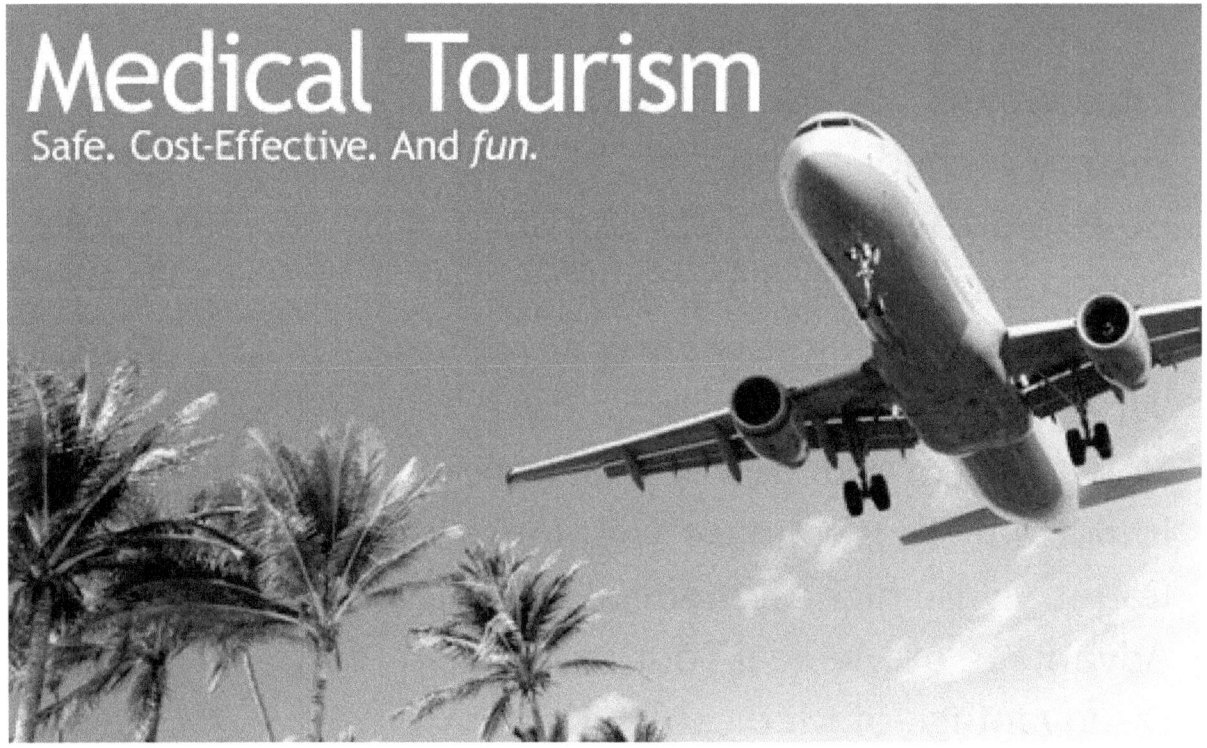

"Health is wealth"- we know this phrase from the childhood. A healthy person can do a lot of work than an unhealthy person. Do you know to maintain a healthy body is not an easy task? Yes, there are too many diseases around us, which always effect to us and make our health weaker. Most often time if new not get rid of this disease, it may cause leads to death. So, it is more important to make better prevention for those persons who are affected. This is the point what I am talking here.

There are many hospitals, clinics, medical institutions around us. There are many doctors, nurses, ward boys- who are always busy to take care of patient.

Some are goods and some are not goods. As this century is a technology dependent century. People can easily get any information from internet and can travel any country easily. So, in case of patient they can also choose better treatment for getting rid from their diseases.

"Medical Tourism" or "Health Tourism" is that plot where people from different countries can choose their better treatment by traveling to other country.

In the past people were used to travel from developing or backward countries to advanced industrialized countries to obtain medical treatment. This was due to the reason that all developing countries did not have technology or expertise to treat some diseases. But from the last decades, this one way process has become two way process of movement of people. Mean to say, people from developed countries are also travelling to developing countries who have established state of the art medical infrastructure over the last couple of decades. This is due to the many reasons. First and the foremost reason is that the medical treatments in developed countries are expensive and all people cannot afford some of the expensive treatments. Second most important reason behind the medical travel of people of developed countries to developing countries is the fact that developing countries offer comparatively cheaper medical treatment facilities to patients.

Another reason people from advanced countries are heading towards developing countries for medical treatment is the problem with the health system of advanced countries. The problem there is long waiting time for treatment due to their free health system. As per estimates of Patients Beyond Borders, in 2013, about 900,000 Americans travelled to other countries to obtain medical treatment. It further estimates global health tourism industry worth $24-$40billion. Now question arises, why the people of developing countries still flying to developed countries, like the UK and the US, to obtain some medical treatment? The reason behind this fact is the technological gap that still exists between developing and developed countries. Some people from developed countries travel to developing countries to obtain organ transplant because the donor of body part is located in that developing country. There are many countries in the world which receive and host millions of medical tourists each year. People travel to other country to obtain treatment of a range of diseases. Later in this book, we will discuss about largest medical tourists hosting countries and major diseases that stimulate the medical tourism around the world.

History of Medical Tourism:

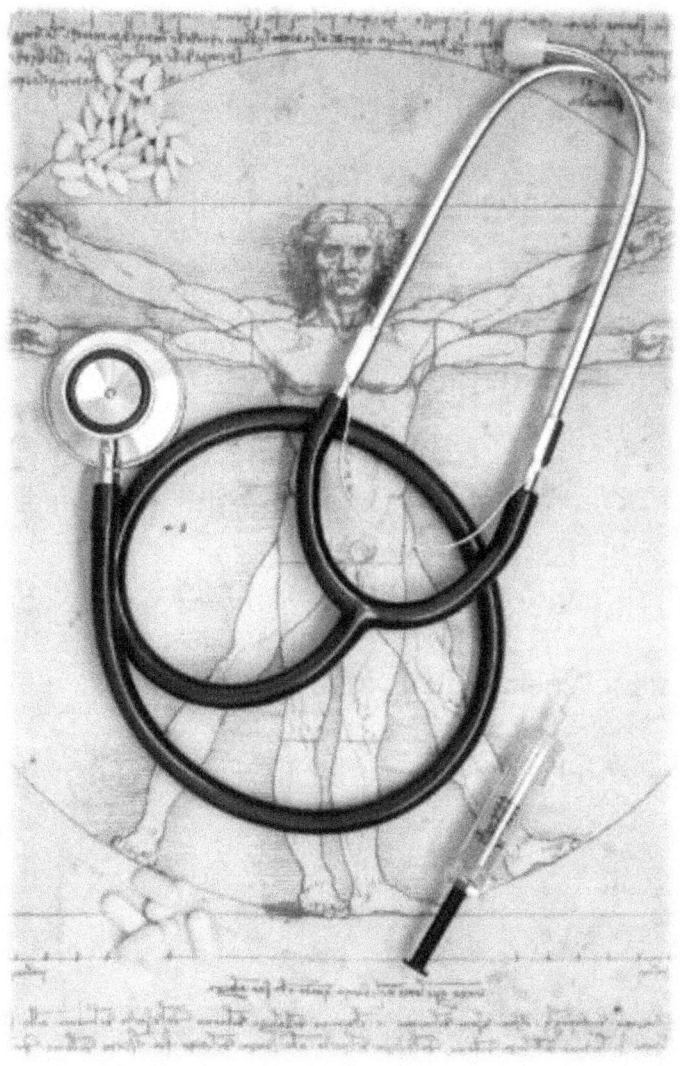

The concept of medical tourism is as old as medicine itself. People have been traveling for centuries in the name of health. They have traveled long distances for health care. Now we will discuss about some of the earliest civilizations which dates back thousands of years:

Earliest Health Complexes:

In 2000 B.C, during the time of Bronze Age, in hill tribes (which are now known as St. Moritz, Switzerland) recognized the health benefits. The benefits were drinking and bathing in iron-rich mineral springs. Bronze Age implements, including votive drinking cups, have also been found around thermal springs in Celtic mineral wells in England, France and Germany.

In 4000 B.C., The Sumerians constructed the earliest known health complexes that were built around the hot springs (mineral water springs).It included with some facilities. The healthcare facilities included elevated temples with flowing pools. Many post-Sumerians understood the healing effects of mineral rich water.

History of Greek Medical Tourism:

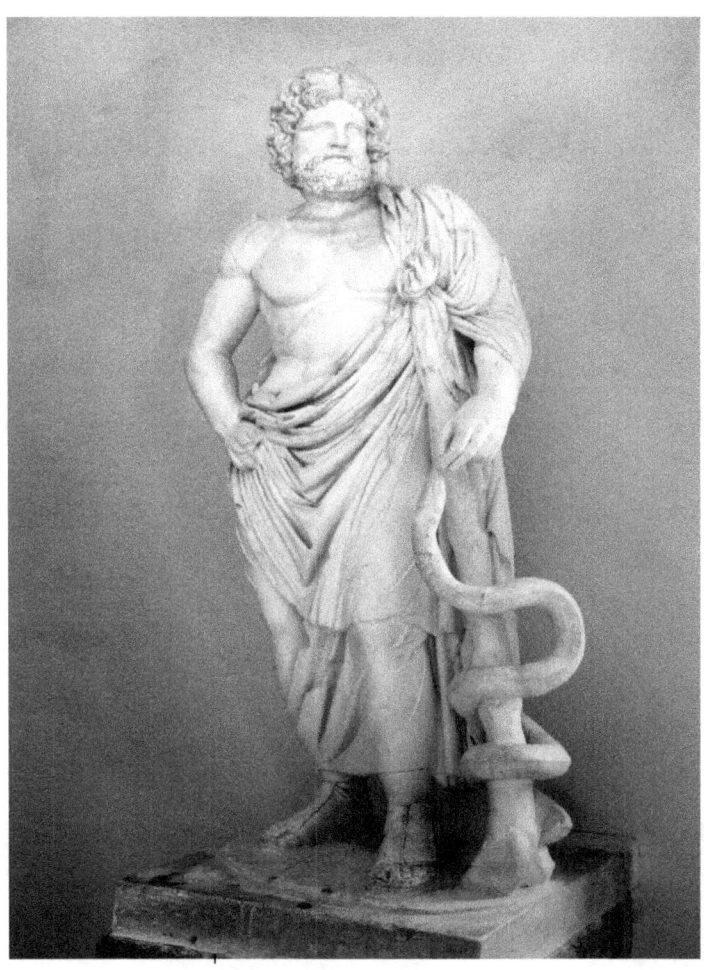

Figure: Asclepius-The God Of Medicine

The ancient Greeks were the first to lay a foundation for a comprehensive medical tourism network. The god of medicine and healing in ancient Greek region "ASCLEPIUS" represents the healing aspect of medical arts. "ASCLEPIUS" erected the asclepiad temples, which became the some of the world first health centers. In between 380-375 B.C., the most famous and large temple was built by "ASCLEPIUS" at Epidaurus in north-eastern Peloponnese. The father of medicine may have begun his career in the Island Of Kos. It was another famous healing temple. The facilities were hot baths, gymnasiums, temples, palestra (exercise area), and a snake farm that was large enough to supply nearby villages. People from all over traveled to these temples to seek cures from their illness like tuberculosis. Patients at the temple were attended to by a retinue of priests, stretcher carriers, and caretakers, before finally being granted an "appointment" with the mighty head priest. Sacrificial payments were made in accordance to the status of the patient – the poor left shoes; Alexander the Great left his breastplate.

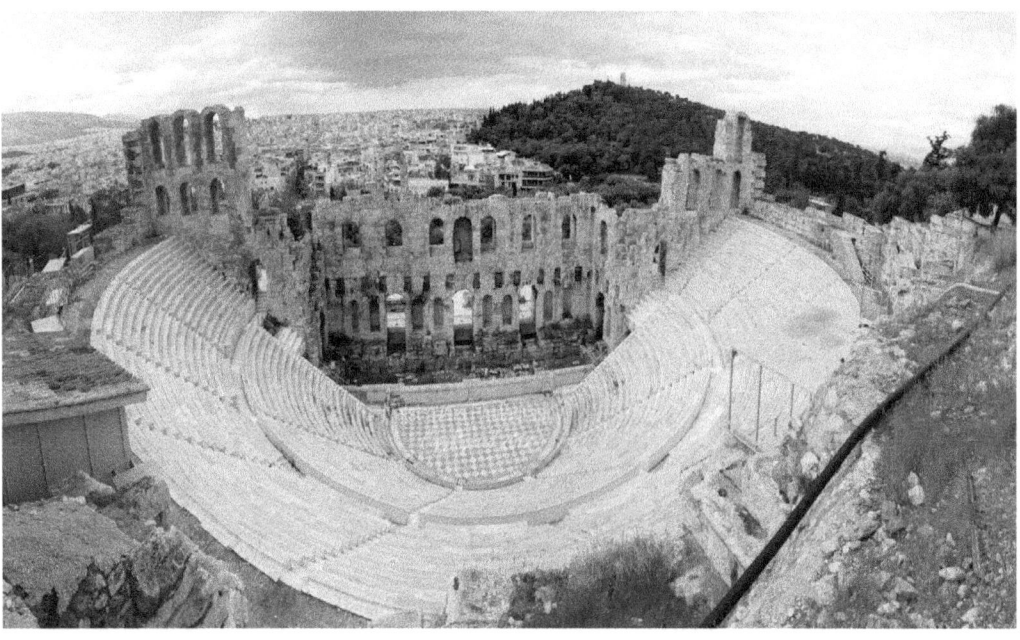

Figure:Present-day remains of the Theater of Dionysus Eleuthereus, Athens

History of Roman Medical Tourism:

When Rome became a global power, they came in existence with the concept of 'THERMAE'. It gained popularity among the elite. 'THERMAE' is hot water baths.

These were the important social networking venues for the most honorable elites. In the time of 16th century, roman was rediscovered by the elites of Europe. They elaborated roman companies. That was included with art galleries, conference halls, lounges, theaters. Some of the houses were up to 3000 patients. The elites of Europe flocked to tourist towns with spas like St.Mortiz, Aachen, and Baden. Bath or Aquae Sulis enjoyed royal patronage. It was famous throughout the known world. It became the center of fashionable wellness. And it became a playground for the rich and famous. After some years the trade market of roman medical centers brought historical changes. They activated trade with Persia, Asia and Africa. Day by day they grew up by receiving Ayurveda message and Chinese acupuncture treatment.

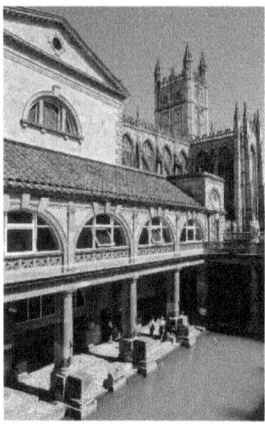

Figure: Roman Baths-Baths Of Caracalla

History of Indian Medical Tourism:

Now a day's India is the global center for medical tourism in Asia. India is offering alternative Ayurveda treatment to plastic surgery. If we look for the history of medical tourism of India, we will see that India was popular with yoga and Ayurveda medicine. As early as 5000 years ago, after the birth of "AYURVEDA'S", the medical travelers flocked to India to seek the benefits of alternative healing methods. Buddhist pilgrimages, yoga, Ayurveda meditation centers were some examples of India's healing arts.

About 2500 years later, with the birth of Buddhism's, India has experienced newly interest of the east. That was about cultural, medical center etc. India is one of the world oldest medical tourism, which is now also serving better treatment for the medical visitors.

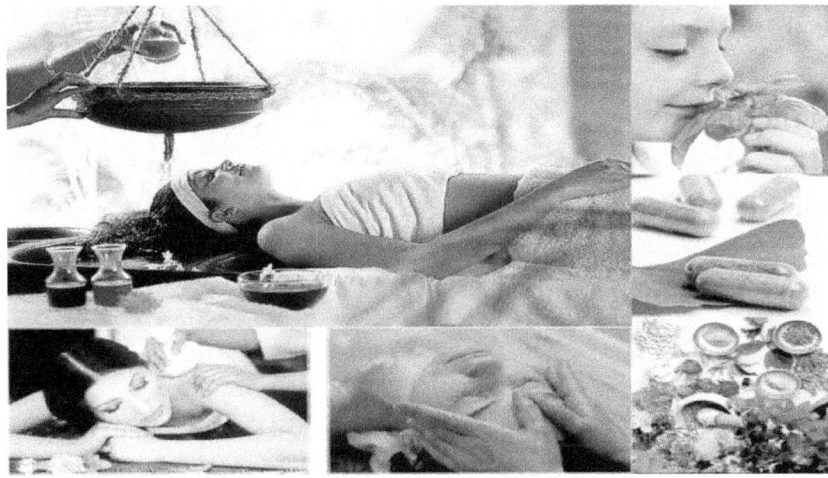

History of Medical Tourism in Europe:

In 1326, a tiny village in east Belgium known as Ville d'Eaux or town of waters became famous through Europe. The iron rich hot springs were discovered within region. Visitors who wanted to get relief of their gout, rheumatism and intestinal disorders, they swarmed to the town of waters. It was hear that the word 'SPA' derived from the roman term 'SALUDE PER AQUA' on health through

Waters was first applied here. Visitors Peter the Great and Victor Hugo visited these wellness resorts.

By the 1720s, aristocrats and wealthy gentlemen flocked to bath for medical treatment. Bath became the first city in England. It obtained funding for the covered sewage system and was ahead of London for several years. Paved roads, elaborated street lighting system, hotels and restaurant ensured comfortable for the medical travelers.

During the 18th and 19th century, several Europeans and Americans liked to travel to the remote areas with spas to prevent various ailments like tuberculosis.

History of Arabic Medical Tourism:

In the 1248 AD. There was a hospital named 'MANSURI', which was situated in Cairo. It was filling with patient capacity of 8000. It contributed a lot in the field of Healing and medicine. This early Islamic civilization included with many facilities like surgery, pharmacy, and separate wards for male, separate wards for female. The hospital treated the patients carefully and made them completely recover from disease. The hospital became a healthcare destination for foreigners regardless of race or religion. There was another hospital in Baghdad, which name was bimaristans. It was also an important healthcare in the history of Arabic medical tourism.

History of Japan Medical Tourism:

Japanese hunters, farmers and fishermen came to small pools of hot water to bath. They thought that by bathing in these rich hot waters, they could relieve from their pain and they could treat arthritic aches. In medieval japan, these hot mineral springs called 'ONSEN'. It became very popular throughout the nation for their healing properties of water. The water was enriched by the surrounding volcanic soil.

After 1000 years, 'ONSEN' became a cultural phenomenon in japan. Many categories of people like tourists, families, businessmen still swim to these revered hot springs like Kyushu.

Now most of the Japanese built big bathtubs and enjoy the onsen experience.

How to Plan Your Medical Tourism:

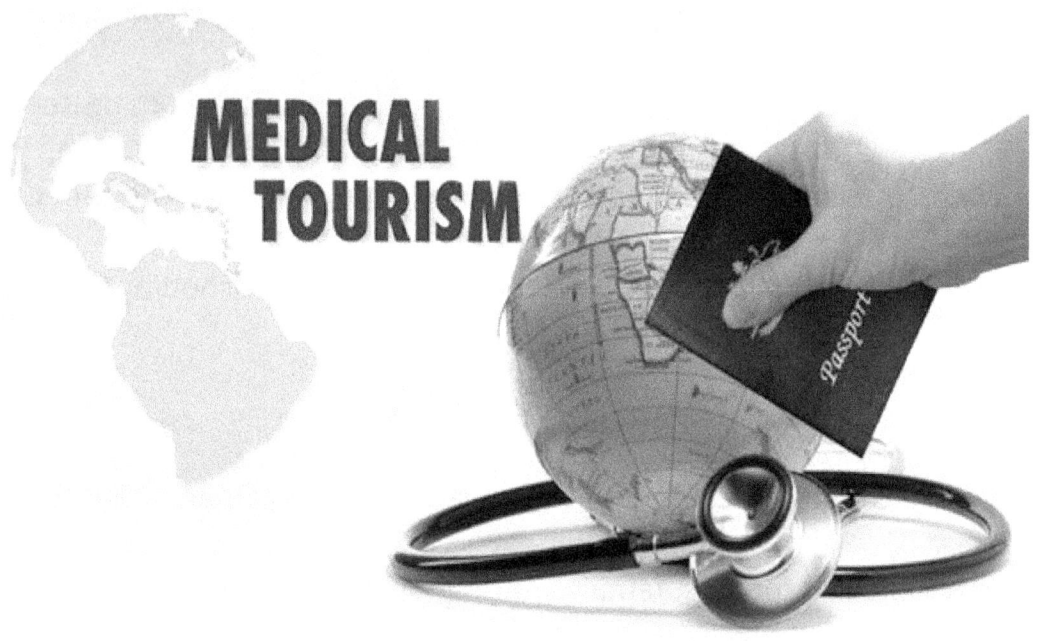

Medical traveling is lucrative. Some travel agencies highlights gorgeous advertisement about medical tourism. But, in reality it is like trap. Sometimes this trap causes the serious harassment to traveler. Without planning there is risk to develop post-surgical complications. Now I will discuss all necessary things that are needed to know before planning a medical tour. You will get all information in this book that you need. Let's see below how you will plan your medical tour:-

Seek Guidance:

Before going for medical tour, you need to collect information about the host country and hospital. You need to gather details on weather, local news, language and hospitality of the country. The hospital where you will visit, you need to know about their reputation, skilled staff, standard of care, affiliation to association etc. And the most important thing is you need to collect all information about the doctor like educational background, work experience, testimonials and success ratio.

Believe Yourself:

Believe yourself and choose a best host country and hospital. Explore more and more. You can contact with travel agency or you can go to internet to explore more. The more research will give you best hospital for you. Later I will discuss medical tourism of different countries. Hope this will help you in this matter.

Don't Be Scarred:

Stay calm and do not be afraid of the operation.

Plan Ahead:

Plan your journey ahead of time. And in the meantime try to judge the selected country and hospital on different qualitative and qualitative criterions.

Set Your Mind To It:

Keep calm and prepared for treatment. Your will is very important in getting well soon.

Email and Internet Searching:

Try to contact with similar patient via phone. If it is not possible to reach that person on phone, contact via email. Moreover, you can also search this kind of people on Facebook, Twitter and LinkedIn.

Questions To Ask To Physician:

It is good to contact your would-be physician and ask everything about future treatment. It would broaden your view if you discuss the before and after elements of treatment to be considered.

Smart Luggage:

If you are travelling alone, then do not take too much luggage with you. It would not be easy to carry too much luggage. Moreover, you do not need too much things of everyday use. The host hospital would provide everything to you. You just can take clothes etc. with you.

Accurately Budget Treatment:

Try to be realistic while planning your medical tour. Do not select cheap deals and cheap hospitals. It is important to be quality oriented. Select a quality travel company to manage your tour. Moreover, select a quality treatment destination.

Important Steps to Plan Medical Tour:

Don't Make Haste:

Give yourself several months' time to plan your medical tour. Especially if you are planning all matters related to medical journey yourself. If it is possible, consult with a consultant or a previous medical tourist to that particular country.

Paperwork and Documentation:

Before you travel make sure you have all the paperwork for your medical journey. Try to confirm the treatment or transplant rates before leaving. What if they ask for more money when they see that you have no other option but to obtain treatment or transplant? So try to document each and every communication with that hospital and that particular doctor.

Travel Distance and Climate Factors:

When you are deciding your health tourism destination you should consider factors such as travel distance, and climate, especially if you are planning an intercontinental travel. If you are in critical situation, then it might not be able to travel to thousands miles away via plane. So in cases of emergencies, consult local doctor first.

Consult Internet and With Previous Patients:

As mentioned in previous chapters, there are a lot of resources on the internet. Use the Internet and Social Media and try to access reliable resource from internet. Try to use reliable resources while you explore websites. Some websites are there just to increase medical tourism not to provide authentic information on the subject.

Language Barriers:

It is related to health and it is important to travel to a country where you can talk to someone in your own language. It is good if English is spoken widely in the destination you have chosen for your medical journey. Al least your destination hospital should have the capacity to provide you English speaking doctors.

Book The Best Quality Hospital and Experienced Doctors:

Before you finalize a hospital, try to research different hospitals, research the medical treatment you need and ask for doctors Resume to check their past related experience. Check on the internet for some testimonies for that hospital and that particular doctor. Also bother to search negative view of the previous patients of that hospital and that particular doctor.

Try To Avoid Crowded Flights Or Places:

Try to book your ticket ahead of time. It is better not to travel during peak holiday seasons. During holiday seasons, you may face delays in flights or hotel or hospital bookings. Also try not to indulge in travel deals and try to book a direct flight to the destination country as long travels are not recommended.

Medical Record and Medical History:

It is important to bring all you medical records with you. Before planning a medical treatment, the doctor there would necessarily need to know you medical history. So accumulate all your medical history related document and reports and put them in your bag in advance. It you do not have previous medical reports or you have lost reports, then try to remember all previous medical history and do consult with your doctor.

What To Do During Stay Abroad:

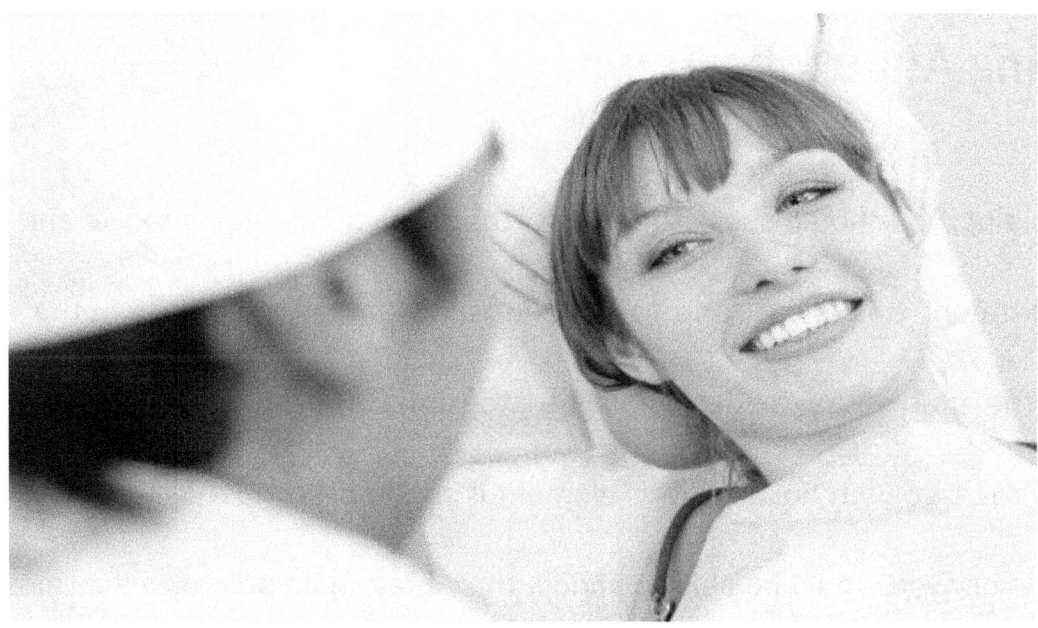

Try to Know About that Country:

It is very important to know about the basics about the country you are

travelling to. In order to avoid troubles, you should try to know the basics of

culture of that country. Moreover, it is pertinent to know about the basics of

the laws you are supposed to follow because ignorance to law is now excused.

General Precautionary Measures:

Do not just rely on tour operators, medical tour consultants and destination

hospitals. You are living in information age where internet offers a lot of resources to help yourself aware enough to decide about your medical treatment tour.

Knowing About the Town:

Before landing, you should check the map of the area you are going to live and obtain treatment. It is so easy and you can find map of every major city of the world on the internet. Even after landing, try to remember the roads and especially roads to your hospital. This element is so important that I case of any emergency you would be able to handle the situation if you are well aware about that place.

Post Treatment Matters:

Strictly follow the pretreatment precautionary measures. The success of your treatment or organ transplant greatly depends upon your current bodily situation. On the other hand, conservatively follow the post treatment precautionary measure to avoid any unwanted problems.

Before Leaving Hospital:

Pay as per agreed terms. Do collect the paper work related to your treatment or transplant. Paper work related to your treatment or transplant may be of use if you need to submit a claim with your insurance company. On the other hand paper work related to your treatment or transplant can serve as proof obtaining consent of donors or organs etc.

Pastime Activities:

It is alright if you hang out if your doctor allows doing so. It is definitely difficult time for you but again do not try to do any irrational act that can cause health risks for you. If you want to visit a place to meet someone or to visit a famous place then before leaving, ask to your doctor. And do not go to crowded places like concerts. If it is possible keep someone with you.

What to Do After Reaching Home:

Family Members and Needs:

Communicate all information related to your medical background and future obligations to keep you safe and sound. Keep at least one family member with you if you have to go out of home.

Starting Old Routines:

Think again and again before starting your old routine works. It is important that you strictly follow the after treatment precautions manual. If you take exercises then consult with your doctor before you start an exercise. If you are a sportsman then do not immediately start play again. Give your body some time to recover from weakness.

Keep in Touch with Local Doctors:

Even after the treatment, keep visiting a local doctor with similar expertise to check your stitches or wounds. There are many examples that after treatment some complications may develop. So it is a good habit to keep visiting your local doctor for proper checkup after treatment.

Take Rest Until You Get Well:

It is right that you have been taking rest for many weeks. But you still need rest if you had a severe treatment or organ transplant. Take time and get rest until you recover from weakness.

Keep Your Paper Work in Safe Place:

Do not waste your all medical history and paperwork of medical treatment and organ transplant. Keep all medical records in safe place for future reference.

What if You Feel Complications? :

Try to keep in touch with the remote doctor that had treated you. Moreover, keep in touch with a local doctor for proper physical checkup. If you feel any kind of complications then immediately contact with remote doctor and local doctor.

After Treatment Precautions:

Try your best to abide by the precautionary guidelines after treatment. Do not eat anything that can harm you. Take some light exercises on daily basis to keep your body in a flow.

How to Make Your Journey Valuable:

It is important to take care of some matters that can make your medical journey valuable. We have discussed the background of medical journey in the Introduction part. Later in we explored further dimensions of Medical Journey. Similarly all related information is discussed in other pages. So it is important to conservatively abide by the rules discussed in this book. All elements discussed in this book are of utmost importance. So it is important to follow all points in letter and spirit. It is better if your insurance company provide health insurance outside of your country.

Selection of a good destination and hospital is not so easy. Take time to select a host country and hospital. Moreover, consider all risks associated with a long travel for medical treatment and organ transplant. If you are not able to travel to a far flung country then try to select a neighboring country. There are also some legal risks associated with medical travel. You may not be able to sure them because it may not be able for you to go there again and file a law suit in case of any service failure. So there are several risks associated with medical journey that must be considered while planning a medical journey.

Important elements to make your journey

Useful:

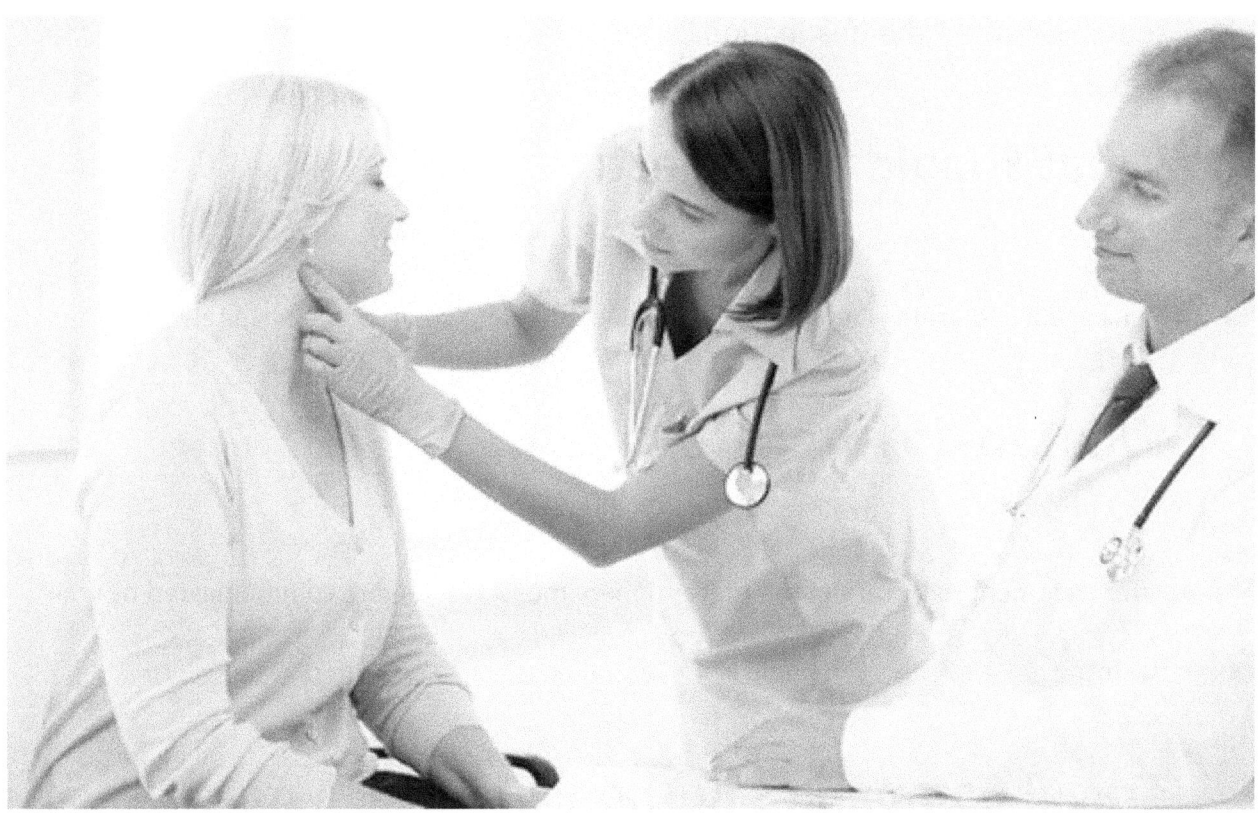

Health Travel Provider:

It is always important to take the help from an expert. So in the case of medical journey it is always desirable to benefit from the expertise of a health travel provider.

In the Meantime:

It was said earlier in this book that you should book your ticket ahead of time of medical treatment. It is important because you can utilize that time in searching about the destination country, hospital and doctor.

What Should You Select:

Think again and again whether you have selected a right country and hospital?

What to do After Treatment:

After treatment, take care of the precautionary measures you are communicated by your doctor.

Travel Companies Responsibilities:

Consider all responsibilities of the travel companies while selecting a travel company. Select a travel company that best facilitate throughout your journey.

Price Oriented or Quality Oriented:

Always try to be quality oriented instead of price oriented. After all, it is a matter of health and one should not compromise on quality.

Countries with Highest Medical Tourism:

Malaysia:

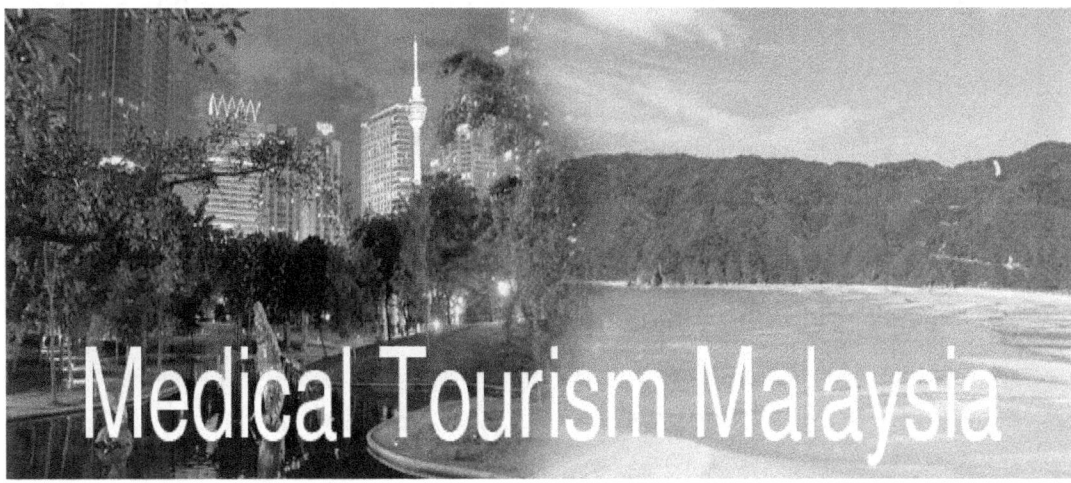

Malaysia is one of the most popular medical tourism places. Over half a million medical tourists, which are maximum from Asia visit Malaysia every year for their medical purposes. The advantage of Malaysia is that English is more widely spoken here. In 2012, Malaysia received 671,727 patients. [Ref: www.medicaltourism.com]

The favorable exchange rate of the US dollar to the Malaysian ringgit (RM) makes the already low cost treatment.

The Island of Penang and Kuala lumpur are leading the Malaysia medical tourism. They both have airlines service from around world, reasonably priced hotel rooms and an excellent public transportation system. The doctors of

Malaysia are either trained in the U.K or the U.S and all of them speak English fluently.

For the help of readers, I am going to give some address and contact number of some well-known hospitals, which are situated in Penang and Kuala Lumpur. So, let's see below:

1) HSC Medical Center:

Address: Pnb Darby Park, Jalan Binjai, 50450 Wilayah Persekutuan, Wilayah Persekutuan Kuala Lumpur, Malaysia

+60 3-2712 0866

2) Institute Jantung Negara (IJN):

Address: 145 Jalan Tun Razak 50400 Kuala Lumpur Malaysia

Phone: +603-2981333

Fax: +603-2982824

Website: http://www.ijn.com.my

Email:info@ijn.com.my

3) Gleneagles Hospital Kuala Lumpur:

Address: 282-286 Jalan Ampang 50450 Kuala Lumpur Malaysia

Phone: +603-4141 3000

Fax: +603-4257 9233

Website: http://www.gleneagleskl.com.my

Email:katrina@gleneagleskl.com.my

4) Penang Adventist Hospital:

Address: 465, Jalan Burma, 10350 Pulau Pinang, Malaysia

Phone :   +60 4-222 7200

5) Sentosa Medical Centre:

Address: 36 Jalan Chemur Damai Complex 50400 Kuala Lumpur Malaysia

Phone: +603-4043 7166

Fax: +603-4043 7761

Website: http://www.sentosa.kpjhealth.com.my/

Email:sentosa@sentosa.kpjhealth.com.my

6) Hospital Lam Wah EE:

Address: Jalan Tan Sri Teh Hwe Lim 11600 Penang, Malaysia

Phone   +60 4-657 1888

Website   http://www.hlwe.com.my

Cosmetic surgery, dental work, dermatology- these are most popular

treatments available in Malaysia. Some hospitals have translators. They can

translate 22 different languages. The cost of medical bill is always reasonable.

For example, a hip replacement at Penang's Lam Wah Ee Hospital is about one third the price of the same operation in the U.S.

Singapore:

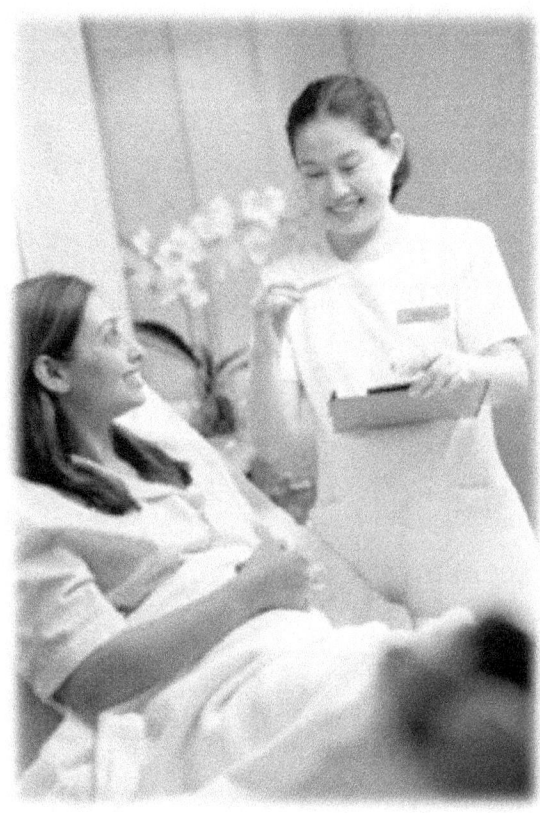

The one of the best medical tourism country is Singapore. This attracts about 200,000 patients every year to receive medical services. A large number of their patients come from Indonesia, China, United States Of America and Europe. The government of Singapore is trying to establish it a regional hub for medical treatments and organ transplants. Last year Gleneagles Hospital in

Singapore was rated as one of the world's top 10 hospitals for medical tourism by Medical Travel Quality Alliance.

Many Singapore hospitals have been accredited by international accreditation agencies like JCI. There are some awesome medical centers in Singapore. Accident and emergency services work 24 hours a day. The doctors are well qualified. The transport systems are quick and efficient.

Some well-known hospitals of Singapore are:

i)Alexandra Hospital

Address: 378 Alexandra Road Singapore 159964.

Tel (General) : 6379-3150,

Email : enquiry@alexhosp.com.sg

Website : http://www.alexhosp.com.sg/

ii) Mount Elizabeth Hospital

Address: 3 Mount Elizabeth Singapore 228510.

Tel (General) : 6737-2666

Tel (24hr/Emergency) : 6735-5000 (ParkwayHealth Patient Assistance Centre Hotline)

Fax : 6734 0518

Email : ppac@parkway.sg

Website : http://www.mountelizabeth.com.sg/

iii) Johns Hopkins Singapore International Medical Centre

Address: 11 Jalan Tan Tock Seng Singapore 308433.

Tel (General) : 6880-2222

Fax : 6880-2223

Email : info@imc.jhmi.edu

Website : http://www.imc.jhmi.edu/

iv) Thomson Medical Centre (TMC)

Address: 339 Thomson Rd Singapore 307677.

Tel (General) : 6250-2222

Tel (24hr/Emergency) : 6350-8812 (24-hour outpatient clinic)

Fax : 6253-4468

Email : contact@thomsonmedical.com, ipc@thomsonmedical.com (international patients

center)

Website : http://www.thomsonmedical.com/

United States of America:

It comes up with no surprise that the medical treatment costs in the US are higher in the world. About 600,000 to 800,000 patients travel to the US for medical treatment. The US has excellent medical care and facilities. Patients don't need to think about quality here. Orthopedic and cardiac surgeries are best and always performed with great care in USA. All doctors are highly professional and qualified. There is no mercy about their service. They are totally strict about their quality.

USA not only best for medical tourism but also best for vacation. There are many theme parks, tourist places. So people can also enjoy there while go for medical purposes.

The transport system is included with air ambulance. All types of health services- operations, treatment, drugs are always available here. You will get treatment of all major diseases. And also you will get major surgeries here.

But it's true that the cost is not reasonable, so sometimes for some serious patients it cannot be destination.

India:

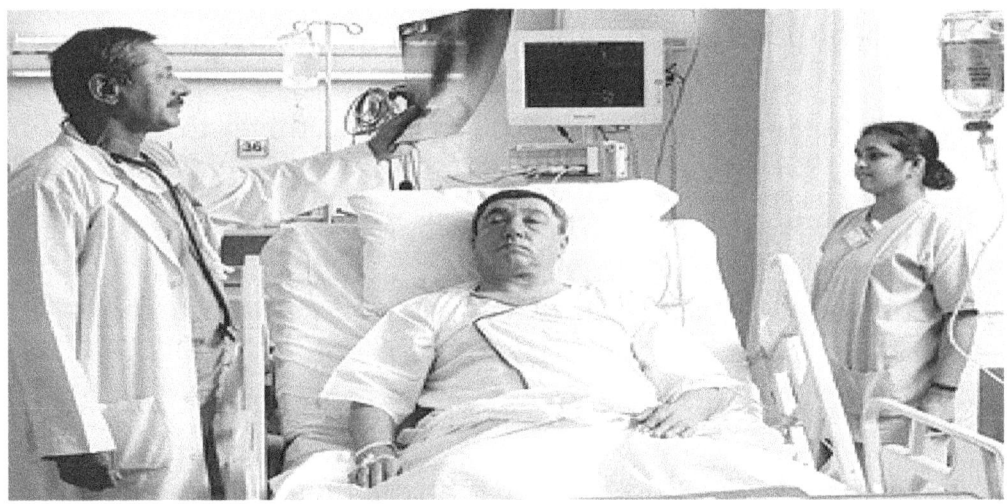

As per estimates of Delloite's report of 2014, medical tourism market is going to reach about $4 billion soon. 250,000 plus patients head toward India every year and the number is growing. Majority of the patients come from neighboring countries, like Bangladesh, Pakistan, Nepal, Bhutan, Myanmar and Sri Lanka. Fertility, Orthopedic, Cardiac and Oncology problems and Organ Transplants are most sought after treatments. A heart valve costs about $15,000 against $150,000 in the U.S, Medical Tourism Resource Guide suggests. The physicians are well trained. The transports and hospital facilities are also good. Heart care has become specialist in India.

India's JCI-accredited hospitals now number 21.

Some of the best hospitals of India are:

i)Apollo Hospitals Group

Apollo Hospitals - Bangalore

Address : 154/11, Opp. IIM B, Bannerghatta Road, Bangalore 560076 India

Apollo Hospitals – Chennai

Address : No. 21, Greams Lane, Off. Greams Road, Chennai 600006 India

Indraprastha Apollo Hospitals

Address : Sarita Vihar, Delhi Mathura Road, New Delhi 110076 India

Apollo Hospitals – Hyderabad

Address : Jubilee Hills, Hyderabad 500033 India

Phone: +91 44 2829.6569, Chennai

Email: enquiry@apollohospitals.com

ii) Fortis Escorts Heart Institute

Address: Fortis Escorts Heart Institute and Research Center Okhla Road New

Delhi, India 110 025

Phone: + 91-99 1099 0342

Email: international.escorts@fortishealthcare.com

iii) Max Healthcare and Super-Specialty Hospitals

Address: 1 Press Enclave Road, Saket, New Delhi, 110017 INDIA

Phone: +91 11 2651 5050

Email: international@maxhealthcare.com

Thailand:

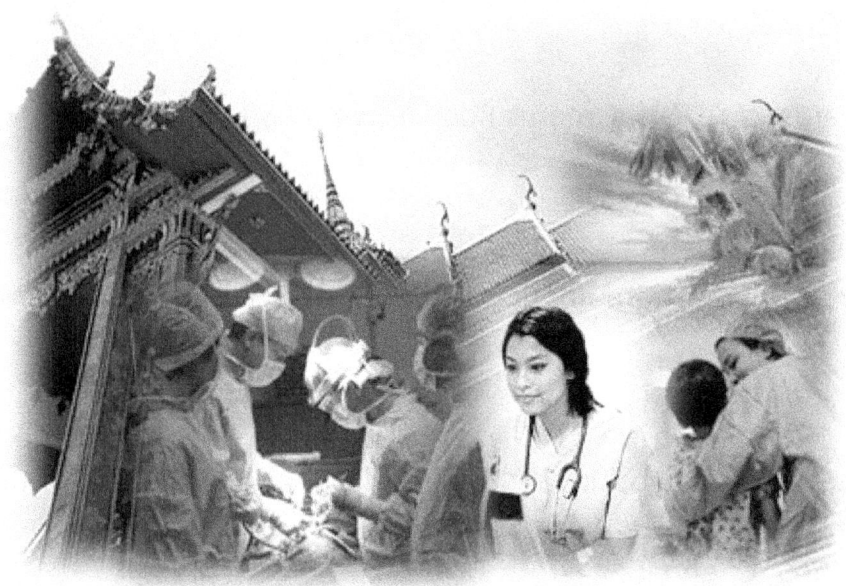

In the early 70s, Thailand became known for sex change operation. In 1980s Thailand came with a largest hospital in South Asia, which name is "Bumrungrad International". It is now the world's most popular destinations for medical tourism. It is located in Bangkok.

According to Patients Beyond borders, it hosted about 1.2 million patients in 2013. Its capital Bangkok is known for its state-of-the-art hospitals. Hospitals at Thailand offer about 50% to 70% less treatment rates than that of the rates of the US hospitals.

Some well-known hospitals are:

i) Bangkok Hospital:

Bangkok hospital was founded in 1972 by a team of doctors, nurses, pharmacists and administering the 100 beds facility. It was the first private medical hospital in Thailand. But today Bangkok hospital is a large group. It has largest hospital operator with 13 network locations throughout Thailand. The hospitals are:

Bumrungrad Hospital and Medical Center (A)

Address : 33 Sukhumvit Soi 3 (Soi Nana Nua), Klong Toey, Bangkok, 10110.
Tel: (02) 667-1000; Fax: (02)667-2525
Website: www.bumrungrad.com

Bangkok Nursing Home Hospital (BNH Hospital)
Address : 9/1 Convent Road, Bangkok, 10500.
Tel: (02) 632-0550,632-0560;
Fax: (02) 632-0577
Website: www.bangkoknursinghome.com

The Bangkok Nursing Home was the first private, non-profit hospital established by expatriates, opening some 100 years ago.

Bangkok General Hospital [A]

Address : 2 Soi Soonvijai 7, New Petchaburi Road, Bangkok, 10320.
Tel.: (02) 310-3000, 318-0066;
Fax: (02) 310-3367
Website: www.bgh.co.th.

Other Private Hospitals Used by Expatriates in Bangkok

Bangkok Christian Hospital (Protestant Mission)

Address : 124 Silom Road, Bangrak, Bangkok, 10500.
Tel.: (02) 233-6981, 634-0560;
Fax: (02) 634-0601
Website : http://www.bangkokchristianhospital.org

Bangkok Mission Hospital (Seventh-Day Adventist Mission) [B/C]

Address : 430 Thanon Pitsanulok (Road), Dusit(near Dusit Zoo), Bangkok, 10300.
Tel.: (02) 282-1100, 281-1422;
Fax: (02) 280-0441
Website : http://www.mission-hospital.com

Paolo Memorial Hospital [B/C]

Address : 670/1 Paholyothin Road, Bangkok, 10400.
Tel.: (02) 271-0227, 271-2460;
Fax: (02) 278-4780

Phayathai 1 Hospital [B]

Address : 364 Sri Ayuthaya Road, Bangkok, 10400.
Tel.: (02) 245-2621-3;
Fax: (02) 642-4468

Phayathai 2 Hospital [B]

Address : 943 Paholyothin Road, Bangkok, 10400.
Tel.: (02) 617-2444;
Fax: (02) 271-2306

Phayathai 3 Hospital (Thonburi)

Address : 207/26 Petchkasem Road, Pakklong, Phasricharoen, Bangkok, 10160
Tel.: (02) 869-1111;
Fax: (02) 869-1119
Website : http://www.phayathai.com

Samitivej Hospital and Medical Center

Address : Sukhumvit Soi 49, Wattana, Bangkok, 10110.

Tel.: (02) 392-0011;

Fax: (02) 391-1290

Website : http://www.samitivijhospitals.com

Samitivej hospital awarded mother & baby friendly hospital by UNICEF and recognized by JCI USA for excellent care in OA Knee, Myocardial infarction, Low back pain, Primary stroke & Lung cancer. It was built in 1979. Samitivej Sukhumvit has grown to be a leading provider of medical healthcare services in Thailand and Southeast Asia. Samitivej Hospital Group has a comprehensive range of facilities and service from cosmetic to tertiary care. It has over 800 doctors, 30 operating theaters and 815 beds. It has long been recognized as a comprehensive facility of choice for locals and tourists. The hospital specialty is Plastic Surgery. Many people from different country come here to get treatment for Plastic Surgery.

St. Louis Hospital (Catholic Mission)

Address : 215 South Sathorn Road, Yannawa, Bangkok, 10120.

Tel.: (02) 675-5000;

Fax: (02) 675-5200

Website : http://www.stlouis.or.th

Ramathibodi University Hospital (Mahidol University)

Address : 270 Rama VI Road, Bangkok, 10400.

Tel.: (02) 246-1073-87;

Fax: (02) 201-1061, 246-0024

Siriraj Hospital (Mahidol University) [D/S]

Address : 2 Prannok Road, Thonburi, Bangkok, 10700.

Tel.: (02) 419-7000, 411-4230; Fax: (02) 411-2429

Website : http://www.si.mahidol.ac.th

Hospital for Tropical Diseases (Mahidol University)

Address : 420/6 Rajavithi Road, Phayathai, Bangkok, 10400.

Tel.: (02) 246-0056, 246-0832, 246-1272;

Fax: (02) 246-8340

This is principally a teaching and research facility.

Prapinklao Naval Hospital (Royal Thai Navy)

Address : 504 Taksin Road, Thonburi, Bangkok, 10600.

Tel.: (02) 468-0116-20;

Fax: (02) 475-2710

Brazil:

Brazil is famous for its common cosmetic treatments. According to Patients Beyond Borders, more than 180,000 patients headed to Brazil last year. It further suggests that Americans can save from 20% to 30% by selecting Brazil for treatment.

Hungary:

Dental patients from neighboring countries like, Germany, Switzerland and Austria prefer Hungary due to inexpensive dental treatments. Cosmetic or restorative dental procedures in Hungary cost between 40 percent and 75 percent in Hungary than that of the U.S.

Turkey:

With proximity with Europe, turkey is attracting huge volumes of Europeans for medical treatments. Hospitals in Turkey specialize in laser treatments in fewer prices than Europe. It hosts about 30,000 patients from 100 countries each year. In Turkey a laser treatment on both eyes starts with 750 Euro ($1,042) including 3 nights stay in hospital.

Israel:

It is also among the major medical treatment patients hosting country. It is a tiny country but has advanced infrastructure and health system. It hosts more than 30,000 medical treatment patients every year.

Iran:

Iran is also attracting significant number of patients around the world. Iran is also a technologically advanced country. Its medical infrastructure is good and it has capacity in its hospitals to host more than 30,000 medical treatment patients from other countries annually.

Advantages of medical Tourism:

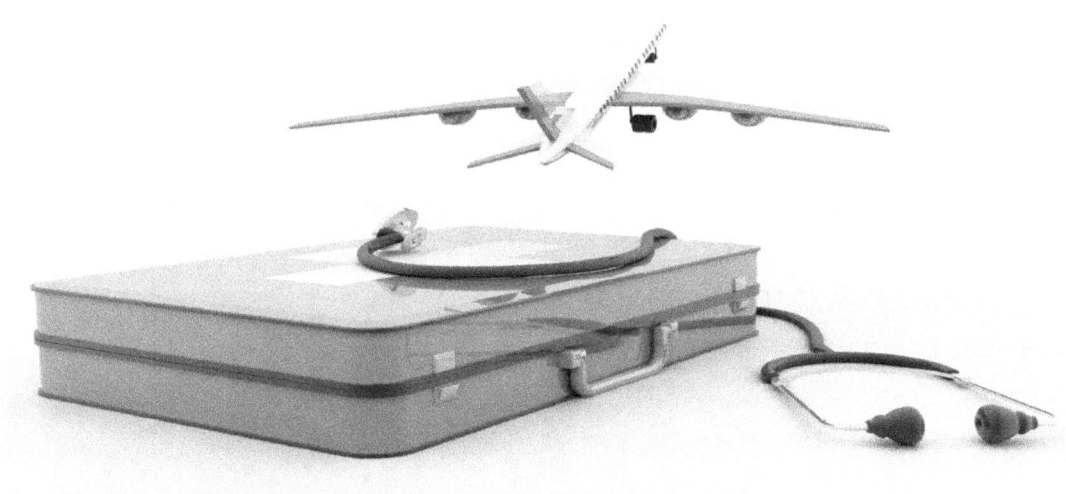

i) The first advantage is better treatment. People don't need to be worried too much. Medical tourism in a best country always ensure better treatment for patient and give back smile in their face again.

ii) In highly developed countries the medical costs are more expensive. Medical tourism gives secure treatment at a reasonable price. The saving ranges are between 30% and 80% of the cost than USA.

iii) The surgical procedures are performed by well-trained physicians. That is a big plus point o0f medical tourism. Many of the doctors and surgeons that offer health care service to international patients, they are most well trained from USA and Great Britain.

iv) You can know upfront estimate of your medical treatment. Most foreign hospitals are willing to provide that. So, you will be able to make a budget.

v) You can enjoy your vacation through medical tourism which will refresh your mind because the countries with medical services are also reputed for their stunning tourism places. So you can get mind blowing excitement by visiting tourism places as well as treatment.

Disadvantages of Medical Tourism:

i) The primary reason is cost. Medical tourism treatment is costly than your local hospital treatment. So sometimes it can't be a destination for serious patients.

ii) Sometimes visa processing, contacting with doctor and maintaining paper work of host country take too much time. So, patient cannot get immediate treatment.

iii) The cultural and language barrier puts medical tourists at a disadvantage.

iv) Sometimes some travel agencies offer big but in return they don't give that offers. In some cases agencies take too much money from patient.

Conclusion

This book is a concise and comprehensive book on medical tourism. At the end, it's time to conclude all discussion in a paragraph. This book starts with introduction to medical tourism. Then we have seen history of medical tourism of different countries and region, how to plan a typical medical tour. We have also discussed important steps to plan a typical medical tour. Then we shed light what should we to during stay abroad & about the steps as what to do after reaching home. Later we have described how to make your journey valuable & about important steps to make a medical journey successful. Finally, last but not least, we can see important statistics about the countries with highest medical tourism. Medical tourism is billions of dollar global industry with millions of patients moving every year to other countries. There are a lot of elements to consider while planning for medical journey. Taking care of you before and after the treatment is very important. After treatment precautionary measures should be strictly followed to ensure your safety. As per estimates of Patients Beyond Borders, in 2013, about 900,000 American travelled to other countries to obtain medical treatment. It further estimates global health tourism industry worth $24-$40billion. Some people from developed countries travel to developing countries to obtain an organ transplant because the donor of body part is located in that developing

country.

The End